101 Natural Hemorrhoid Treatments

Treat & Cure Piles
Hemorrhoids Pain Relief
Haemorrhoids Remedies A to Z

D1714359

Lindsey James

Pink Parachute

Sussex, England

ISBN 978-1-907619-00-7

Introduction

Hemorrhoids are a pain!

However, if you are a sufferer, you're not alone. Estimates are that half of us develop hemorrhoids by the age of 50. They are also common amongst pregnant women.

Hemorrhoids, otherwise known as piles or haemorrhoids, are the swelling and inflammation of veins in the rectum and anus. There are two types.

External hemorrhoids are those that are outside the end of the anal canal They are often painful, and the skin irritation can lead to the desire to itch.

Internal hemorrhoids occur inside the rectum. Because the area lacks pain receptors, they are not usually painful, and you may not be aware that they exist. The first symptom is often bleeding. Untreated, they can become prolapsed (pushed outside) or strangulated (no blood supply).

Hemorrhoids are often caused by:

- Constipation, or sometimes diarrhoea. Trying to defecate too often, particularly straining, can lead to hemorrhoids.
- Obesity. Extra weight on the pelvic area, together with the poorer muscle tone and posture associated with overweight people cause the problems.
- Pregnancy. The extra weight, together with greater strain during bowel movements often bring on hemorrhoids.

A high fiber diet, sufficient exercise and keeping weight down are all vital prerequisites to combatting hemorrhoids. These, together with other important issues are covered in this book, together with other herbal, homeopathic Chinese and Ayurvedic (traditional Indian) treatments.

I hope you find it useful. There are plenty of alternatives and you should hopefully find relief from one or more treatments that suit you.

Important

It is important not to undertake any treatment without the agreement of your medical practitioner. You need them to make sure that it is hemorrhoids that you're suffering from - it could be a fissure, an abscess, or something else. And you need them to sanction your treatment.

Many treatments are not suitable for everyone - particularly if you're taking other medicines or suffer from problems like high blood pressure, or you are pregnant.

Homeopathic treatments are often based on toxic substances that can prove dangerous, even fatal, if not taken under medical supervision.

1
Acupuncture

cupuncture stimulates discrete points of the body by inserting tiny needles into specific acupoints in the skin. These are situated on meridians, along which *qi*, a life energy flows.

It is often the ears that are treated for hemorrhoids as the nerves in the ear are believed to relate directly with the lower rectal, anal region.

The idea is to eliminate the stagnation of blood flow along the nerve path which leads to the pain in the anus.

Typically, the needles are left in place for 30 minutes for each treatment, with the needle being rotated 300 times per minute every 5 minutes.

Some soreness and numbness is often felt, particularly in the lower leg, but many patients start benefitting from hemorrhoid relief after several days of treatment.

As with all treatments in this book, do obtain approval from your medical practitioner before trying it, as it may not be suitable for you.

2
Alfalfa

Alfalfa is also known as Lucerne. It is a perennial flowering plant of the pea family that grows in temperate climates.

As it is particularly rich in both fiber and protein it is one of the most important feeding crops for dairy cattle. Most hemorrhoid sufferers, however, derive the greatest benefit from applying the juice to inflamed piles. You can find the substance in health food and homeopathy outlets.

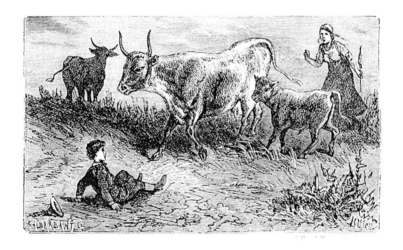

Or, depending on where you live, in a nearby field of cows. But that is not advised - you may not be sure enough of what you are eating - or indeed, sure of the cattle!

3
Aloe Vera

Aloe Vera is also known as medicinal aloe. It grows in arid areas, particularly in Africa. It contains anthraquinones, polysaccharides, mannans and lectins and is widely used as a herbal medicine for healing, soothing and moisturising.

Aloe Vera gel can be applied directly to relieve pain and soothe the burning sensation.

Alternatively the juice can be drunk and is used for relieving constipation and hemorrhoids.

4
Alumroot

Alumroot is a herbaceous perennial plant native to North America.

It is an astringent herb with antiseptic properties that was used by Native Americans to aid digestive difficulties. The root is available from herbalist outlets and can either be ingested or applied externally.

5
Amla

Amla is a deciduous tree, also known as the Indian gooseberry.

Because of its ability to reduce inflammation and tackle constipation it has been widely used for thousands of years in Indian Ayurvedic medicine. It is described in ancient texts as *promoting longevity and inducing nourishment.*

6
Apis Mellifica

Apis Mellifica is a homeopathic remedy made from honeybees.

Ideally, just the venom sac of the honeybee is used, or

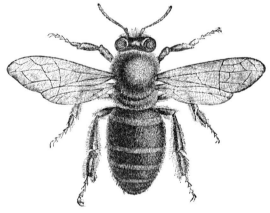

even the actual sting venom - *Apis venenum purum*. This is however, more expensive than the basic *Apis mel* which uses the whole bee.

It is available in ointments, tablets and pellets for fast relief. It can be particularly beneficial if the area is bright red burning and itching.

7
Apple Cider Vinegar

A pple Cider Vinegar has been used for many generations to help prevent infection and the growth of bacteria and it is also known for its anti-inflammatory properties.

Simply soak a cotton ball in apple cider vinegar and apply it to the external hemorrhoids two to three times a day. The intense itching should immediately feel better and in two or three days the swelling should recede and the hemorrhoid will be just about gone within a week.

You can also drink it to help reduce swelling and internal hemorrhoids that you cannot access with a cotton ball.

Insight:
Ayurvedic Medicine

Ayurvedic medicine is an ancient traditional medicine native to the Indian subcontinent. The earliest mention is over 2000 years ago, but many scholars believe a form has been used for over 3000 years.

It is now practised throughout the world and classed as an alternative medicine in the West.

The literal translation from Sanskrit is *The Science of Life*. The basic principle is that everything, including the human body, is composed of the five great elements - earth, water, fire, air and ether. It aims to create a balance of the three great energies - vata (air in space, ie wind), pitta (fire in water -ie bile) and kapha (water in earth, ie phlegm).

Everyone has a unique combination of these balances (Doshas) that needs to be corrected.

8
Banana

Mash a ripe banana in one cupful of milk. Eat this mashed mixture three to four times a day.

It can help stop the painful symptoms of the piles, but is a long-term remedy. Alternatively, make a thick gruel of rice in buttermilk, to which a mashed ripe banana has been added.

9
Barberry

Barberry (Berberis is the Latin genus) is a low growing shrub with long spiny shoots that grows in both temperate and subtropical regions. Because of the spines they are difficult to harvest, but the berries are edible with a very sharp flavour and are rich in vitamin C.

The fruits can be used much like other berries and made into a jam or juice. It is a laxative and can soften stools. Or the root bark can be boiled in distilled water and then used as an astringent with antiseptic properties to clean the anal area.

10
Bilberry

B ilberry, otherwise known as *Vaccinium myrtillus* is a low growing shrub commonly found growing wild in Europe.

It has exceptionally high levels of anthocyanin (dark blue) pigments which are, according to folk medicine, useful in treating hemorrhoids.

11
Bioflavonoids

B ioflavonoids are also known as vitamin P and citrin. They are widely distributed in plants fulfilling many functions.

Bioflavonoids produce yellow, red, and blue pigmentation in petals which protects plants from attacks by microbes and insects. They are also beneficial to animals that eat the plants due to their ability to help the body deal with allergens, viruses, and carcinogens.

In humans they are believed to strengthen vein walls

and reduce inflammation. A good source is citrus fruits, so including more fruits such as oranges, and grapefruits in your diet can help.

Alternatively green tea, red wine, and dark chocolate also contain high quantities.

Side effects are rare, and it is a particularly safe option for pregnant women. There is a product called Daflon, available from health food shops that contains a high quantity of bioflavonoids.

12
Bowel Training

S training can severely aggravate hemorrhoids. Ideally have a daily schedule to go to the toilet and thereby train your body to evacuate regularly.

If you're not able to go, don't sit on the toilet for long periods -- five minutes should be more than sufficient. Also if you feel the urge to go then do so as soon as you can and don't strain.

The posture on the toilet is also important.

Until very recently in man's evolution we squatted. This is a more natural position to help evacuation. Because it is also more uncomfortable, it has the added advantage of helping reduce the time on the toilet.

You can improve your posture by putting a footstool in front of the bowl and resting your feet on it whilst sitting. If a footstool isn't possible then just bend forward with your elbows resting on your knees.

These methods will help an evacuation to take place with much less strain and therefore a reduced chance of developing hemorrhoids.

If you suffer from constipation then some of the remedies in this book may help.

You can also try some gentle deep breathing whilst on the toilet and gently rocking from side to side and back to front with your torso as well.

13
Bromelain

Bromelain is an enzyme found in the pineapple. Bromelain extract typically contains two different Bromelain enzymes together with peroxidase acid and calcium.

It works by blocking metabolites that inflame the tissues on the anus and is also often used to reduce the inflammation of sports injuries

.

14
Burdock Roots

B urdock is a group of biennial thistles native to Europe and Asia.

Don't try and pick Burdock yourself as you might get dermatitis from touching any of the plant that is above the ground.

However an ointment is available from health shops. It can provide relief from inflamed itching and painful hemorrhoids.

15
Butchers Broom

B utchers broom is a herb known as *Ruscus aculeatus*. It is also commonly called Box Holly, Knee Holly, and Sweet Broom.

It has its name as it was once used by butchers to clean their chopping blocks.

Butchers broom is believed to have anti-inflammatory properties that can improve vein structure and shrink swollen hemorrhoids. It can be particularly useful in patients with poor circulation and can either be applied as an ointment or taken internally in a capsule.

It can also be made into a tea, although it is rather bitter, so most people add a sweetener.

Although Butchers Broom can be beneficial for some people, be very careful with it. It is not recommended for anyone taking other drugs, pregnant or nursing women, or people with high blood pressure.

16
Buttermilk

After being prepared from cow's milk, add some peppercorns, rock salt, and ginger and drink twice a day. This can reduce the pain.

17
Calendula

C alendula is a homoeopathic ointment made from the flower of the Marigold plant. It is particularly useful for open wounds, ulcers, and hemorrhoid bleeding that won't stop. Unfortunately it is not generally available in the United States.

18
Cascara

C ascara, otherwise known as Bearberry, Buckthorn, Chitticum or *Rhamnus purshianus* is a large shrub native to western North America.

It was known by the Native Americans for its laxative properties and can counteract constipation and thereby hemorrhoids. It is available from health stores and herbalists.

19
Catechu

Catechu is an extract of the Acacia tree. It is made by boiling the wood in water and reducing the liquid. It is known for its astringent properties in Ayurvedic medicine.

20
Cayenne Pepper

This might sound strange but this can work. Mix one quarter a teaspoon of cayenne pepper in half a pint of water and drink it. Do this twice a day but only for a few days as it can aggravate the stomach.

21
Camomile

Camomile is a common name for several daisy like plants. When made into a tea it is commonly used to help with sleep and is often served with lemon or honey. It is an anti-inflammatory that soothes irritated tissues, reducing redness and itching. It can be used for hemorrhoids by cooling a camomile tea in the refrigerator and then applying it to the hemorrhoids. Alternatively a camomile ointment can be applied directly.

22
Camphor

C amphor is extracted from the wood of the Camphor tree, a large tree found in Japan and south east Asia.

In herbal treatment camphor can be applied topically using a 1% solution. It has anaesthetic and antifungal properties.

23
Cleansing

I t is good practice to use a mild soap together with plenty of water to clean your anus after using toilet paper. Rather than run the risk of fingernails scratching it is better to use a soft cloth. Alternatively you can purchase medicated wipes that work well. Try to avoid any repeated wiping with toilet paper.

24
Coconut Oil

If the pain from your hemorrhoids is particularly bad apply some coconut oil to the affected parts. It should bring short-term relief, but should not be used for any lengthy period.

25
Collinsonia Canadensis

This is a medicinal herb from the mint family, native to the Americas. Common names include Canada Horsebalm, Horseweed and Stone Root. It provides relief from an itching anus, hemorrhoids and constipation and is used in homeopathic medicine.

26
Comfrey

Comfrey is a medicinal herb with a black root and large, hairy, bell shaped leaves native to Europe. It contains allantoin, a cell proliferant that aids the body in replacing cells.

It can be applied externally as a paste or a lotion to aid the healing process after the initial treatment of hemorrhoids.

27
Cranesbill

C ranesbill is the name given by herbal medecine practitioners to geraniums. *Geranium maculatum* is the wild geranium that Native Americans used to aid digestion.

In herbal medicine the root and rhizome is used as a poultice. It has astringent properties.

28
Cumin Seeds

C umin originated in the Middle East and is a herbaceous annual plant of the parsley family.

Take some seeds and roast them over in a frying pan. Mix one tablespoon of these seeds with the same amount of seeds that haven't been roasted. Crush and then mix thoroughly. Stir one quarter of the mixture into a glass of water and drink once per day. This can provide significant relief for hemorrhoids.

29
Dong Quai

D ong quai, otherwise known as female ginseng or *Angelica Sinensis* is a herb native to China.

Its dried root is known as Chinese angelica in Chinese medicine and is widely used to treat disorders of the circulatory system as well as gynaecological ailments, fatigue and it also said to be an aphrodisiac.

It has analgesic, anti-inflammatory and sedative properties.

30
Drying the Area

T he moister the anus is, the more likely it is to suffer from irritation and infection. Pat it dry after bathing or swimming and then sprinkle it with baby powder.

31
Eggplant

The eggplant it is also known as the aubergine or brinjal. It is a berry native to India.

An ointment needs to be prepared by mixing 100g of animal fat and 40g of chopped eggplant. Cover and place in a low oven for five or six hours. Strain and then store in the fridge. This can be applied to hemorrhoids to reduce inflammation.

32
Elder Leaves or Flowers

Elder is a tree native to North America and Europe. Parts of the varieties of elder with blue/black berries have been used medicinally for centuries. Hippocrates mentioned them as long ago as 400BC and Native Americans were also aware of their benefits in treating skin disorders.

The most common treatment for hemorrhoids is to use the leaves or flowers to brew into a tea.

33
Epsom Salts

E psom salts are known as magnesium sulphate and have been used for many centuries for treating abscesses and boils. They can soothe aches and pains. You can soak in a bath with added Epsom salts or mix with water and rub onto the affected areas.

34
Exercise

E xercise improves circulation, which helps the swollen blood vessels. Moderate aerobic exercise is good. If it is too vigorous it can increase blood pressure too much and make things worse. A brisk walk for around half an hour each day will help.

In addition it is beneficial to improve your pelvic floor muscles. These are the muscles that you use to stop the flow of urine whilst urinating.

A good exercise is to inhale whilst tightening these muscles and hold this position for 10 seconds whilst exhaling slowly. Repeat this for five minutes twice daily.

35
Euphorbia or Spurge

E uphorbia is a genus of plant that is one of the most diverse, being found in tropical, sub tropical and temperate zones throughout most of the world. Its members are sometimes called Spurges.

Euphorbia prostata is believed by some to be a very effective treatment for hemorrhoids.

36
Fenugreek

F enugreek is grown primarily in India, but also throughout the world. Its leaves are used as a herb, whilst its seeds are a spice.

The seeds are used in traditional Chinese medicine where they are known as Hu Lu Ba.

And the leaves are also known for improving digestion and relieving constipation and hemorrhoids.

37
Fiber

Fiber is beneficial to the body generally. It is particularly useful for treating hemorrhoids as it can soften stools and increase their bulk, which helps to reduce straining.

Fiber intake can be increased by switching to wholemeal bread, more fruit & vegetables, and a high fiber cereal for breakfast. You can also purchase products such as powdered Flax seeds or psyllium husks.

It is important however to introduce extra fiber reasonably gradually and also to increase your consumption of water as otherwise constipation may get worse.

38
Figs

Figs can play a useful role in improving the regularity of bowel movements. You can soak figs in water overnight, perhaps with apricots dates or raisins as well and then eat the figs twice daily. You can also drink the water that they stood in.

39
Garlic

Gently beat a clove of garlic, then cut the end off and wring out the juice. Swab the garlic juice onto external hemorrhoids once per day for a week.

40
Ghee

Ghee, also known as clarified butter is made mixing unsalted butter with water and then boiling away all the liquid. The clarified butter is then spooned off. Ghee is almost entirely saturated fat. If you take 4 teaspoons of ghee daily, together with a high fiber diet, you should find that stools will be easier to pass.

41
Ginger

Mix about half a teaspoonful of ginger juice, half a teaspoonful of lime juice, half a teaspoonful of mint juice, and one tablespoonful of honey together. Take this once per day.

42
Ginkgo

G inkgo, with a Latin name of *Ginkgo biloba* is a very large tree with long branches and deep roots. It is disease resistant, with some trees believed to have lived for 2500 years. It is the national tree of China.

Gingko extract is believed to help the blood flow and has been used as a hemorrhoid treatment for many centuries.

43
Goats Milk

T his remedy is particularly useful for bleeding hemorrhoids. Let a quarter of a litre curdle overnight. Then add the same quantity of carrot juice. Mix together and drink. You can also obtain goats milk yoghurt that you can mix with freshly chopped carrots and take regularly.

44
Goldenseal

G oldenseal is a perennial herb native to North America. Herbalists use it to treat hemorrhoids due to its anti-inflammatory, antiseptic and astringent properties.

45
Gotu Kola

G otu Kola is the name given to the medicinal herb *Centella asiatica* It is used in Ayurvedic and Chinese medicine, as it relaxes the aorta and veins, allowing blood to flow better and increasing capillary strength. It also helps the skin heal.

46
Gourd

G ourds are related to pumpkins. Gourd juice is a common drink in China with a distinctive smokey taste. Drinking this juice together with buttermilk can relieve hemorrhoids.

47
Graphites

This is a crystalline form of carbon with a smooth greasy texture. It is available from homoeopathic outlets and is often called back lead. It is particularly useful if the anal area is sore and itchy.

48
Haritaki

Haritaki is a herbaceous plant used in Ayurvedic medicine, otherwise known as Chebulic Myrobalan, Ink Nut or *Terminalia chebula*. It only lacks one (salty) of the six tastes that describe treatments. It has a very similar effect to Amla, but this has a heating effect, whereas Amla cools.

49
Hawthorn

Hawthorn is a large genus of shrubs and small trees. The Chinese Hawthorn, *Crataegus pinnatifida* is used in

Chinese medicine. Its dried fruits are called Shanzha and are used as a digestive aid. Its Japanese counterpart, *Crataegus cuneata*, and the species known as *Crataegus laevigata* are used in a similar way.

50
Hemorrhoid Cushion

This can be useful for some sufferers. A hemorrhoid cushion is usually an inflatable rubber ring that you sit on. It works by removing or minimising contact between the sitting surface and the hemorrhoid.

It may also relieve the pressure of the cheeks on any prolapsed hemorrhoids. Alternatively a soft cushion or pillow may help.

51
He Shou Wu

He Shou Wu, otherwise known as Hoshouwu, Knotweed or *Polgonum multiflorum* is a Chinese herb.

When ingested it has a laxative effect, relieving constipation. It also tones the kidneys.

Insight:
Homeopathy

Homeopathy is a type of alternative medicine that believes that you should treat like with like. It uses heavily diluted preparations of substances which, in slightly greater concentration would cause symptoms similar to those being suffered by the patient - and an even greater dose could prove to be poisonous, even fatal.

It has been practised for over 200 years and its acceptance as a valid means of treatment varies widely from country to country.

Homeopaths are guided by the mental and physical state of the patient in deciding on the treatment.

The dilution is often so great that none of the original preparation remains. It has been proposed that water has a memory that allows the resultant treatment to work when it seems to be wholly water.

It is generally regarded as safe, despite highly toxic substances forming the base of many preparations.

52
Horse Chestnut

This is very similar to butchers broom. It can be particularly useful when poor circulation is a major contributing factor and can increase the strength and tone of the veins.

It can be either applied externally or made into a tea or eaten in capsule form. Some parts of the horse chestnut are dangerous to eat and there can be rare side effects including kidney and liver damage so only take under appropriate supervision.

53
Horsetail

Horsetail, otherwise known as Bottlebrush or *Equisetum arvense* is one of the oldest surviving plants from prehistoric forests, with some of the species resembling horse's tales.

The young stems are cooked and eaten in Japan routinely, being similar to asparagus. The Romans also used horsetail in this way, and also made it into a tea. Its main use is to help rebuild connective tissue.

It can be ingested by mixing a tablespoon of horsetail in a litre of water and drinking or applied as a cream externally.

54
Ice

E veryone knows that ice packs can reduce swelling. As you can imagine it is not easy to apply an ice pack to veins resulting from hemorrhoids, particularly as many doctors advise keeping a towel between ice and one's skin.

However ice packs can be applied externally if shaped correctly and can provide welcome relief.

55
Ignatia

T his is from a tree found in the Philippines and China. It is a homoeopathic option, and only small doses should be taken under supervision.

It is particularly useful for hemorrhoids that are giving you stabbing pains.

56
Jambul

Jambul is otherwise known as Rose Apple and is an evergreen tropical tree native to southern and southeastern Asia.

The Ayurvedic Indian holistic healing method advises eating jamun or jambul fruit with salt each morning for three months.

57
Japanese Pagoda Tree

Japanese Pagoda Tree (*Styphnolobium japonicum*) is one of the small genus of small trees and shrubs in the pea family.

Despite its name it is native to China and was introduced into Japan a few hundred years ago.

It reduces bleeding, and improves veins.

58
Keep a Healthy Weight

If you are overweight you are lifting your excess weight up each time you stand, walk, or run.

And whilst sitting the weight of your upper body is bearing down on your anal region and it may well aggravate hemorrhoids.

59
Lavender Oil

Lavender oil can ease the pain of hemorrhoids by being applied directly to the affected area.

60
Lemon

Squeeze the juice of a lemon into some hot milk and drink.

61
Loose Clothing

Tight fitting clothing, particularly underwear, can aggravate hemorrhoids because it can restrict blood flow and put extra pressure on the hemorrhoids.

62
Mango Seeds

Mango seeds help the digestive system as they increase peristalsis, which improves evacuation. Seeds can be taken from ripe mangoes and dried. After being ground into a fine powder this can be used in the future by taking 2g of powder with honey twice a day for a couple of months.

63
Mullein

Mulleins are of the genus *Verbascum*, in the figwort family. They are native to Asia and Europe.

Verbascum thapsus is used as a herbal remedy to provide soothing relief from pain.

64
Mustard

Some people have found that eating mustard mixed with dairy products has eased the pain of hemorrhoids.

You could try grinding some black mustard to a powder and mixing this in to a bowl of yoghurt. Alternatively mix the ground black mustard into some goats milk.

65
Myrrh

Myrrh is a dark red resinous substance made from tree sap, primarily *Commiphora myrrha*, native to Somalia, Yemen and Ethiopia.

It is classified in Chinese medicine as being suitable for moving blood and thus hemorrhoid relief. It is also used in Ayurvedic and herbal medicines.

Mix 1 teaspoon of powdered myrrh with 1 teaspoon of

water to make a thick paste. Apply to the affected area and leave it there for an hour or two to relieve the pain and swelling.

66
Neem

Neem is a tree of the mahogany family. In India the tree is called various names including divine tree, heal all, nature's drugstore, and village chemist.

It is known in Ayurvedic medicine for its antibacterial, anti-inflammatory and pain relieving properties. An extract of Neem applied externally can soothe external hemorrhoids.

67
Nitricum Acid

Commonly called Nitric Acid, it is used in homeopathic medicine for constipation, and pain relief.

68
Nux Vomica

This is a medium-sized tree native to India. It is highly poisonous, with most parts of the tree containing the alkaloids Strychnine and Brucine.

It is used in homoeopathic medicine to treat painful hemorrhoids and chronic constipation.

69
Oil Treatment

Aromatherapists often recommend adding 1 or 2 drops of cypress, juniper, lavender or rosemary oil to vegetable oil and applying it to the affected area.

70
Onion

This is supposed to be a fast working remedy, although it can give you rather bad breath! Chop one small onion and mix with about three tablespoons of sugar. Eat twice a day.

Alternatively crush the onion and drink the onion juice, again mixed with sugar, twice a day for a month.

71
Paeonia Officinalis

Commonly called Peony, it is used in homeopathic medicine to relieve anal itching and the burning pain that can be suffered after defecating.

72
Papaya

Papayas contain an enzyme called papain and can reduce inflammation, helping to provide hemorrhoid relief. They are also a good source of fiber.

73
Pasque Flower

The Pasque flower is a deciduous perennial that grows in northern Europe and North America. Pasque refers to Easter/Passover as it flowers at that time of year. It is highly toxic but is used in homoeopathic medicine for hemorrhoids that itch and also have sharp stabbing pains.

74
Passion Fruit

A paste made from 3g of fruit extract mixed with water can be applied to the affected area to soothe and relax the skin.

75
Pilewort

Pilewort has been used to treat hemorrhoids. It is now often called celandine and is a low growing plant indigenous to Asia and Europe.

It was named after piles, both because it was a cure, and also because the knobbly tubers resemble hemorrhoids.

It is a quick acting astringent that tones the blood vessels, and stops bleeding but can be dangerous, so, as with all treatments, should only be tried under medical supervision. It can be added to baths and is widely available in pharmacies.

76
Pomegranate

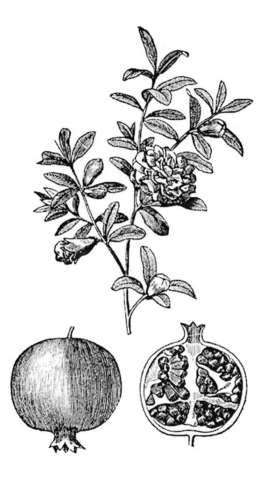

P eel a pomegranate and boil the peelings in water. Drink the water twice daily.

Or saturate a cotton ball with the juice and dab the affected area.

77
Psyllium

P syllium is the common name for the annual herb that is a member of the genus *Plantago* that grows in Europe and the Indian subcontinent.

The seeds have a high fiber content and are used to make high fiber cereals. They are also used in such commercial products as Fybogel in the UK, Bonvit in Australia and Metamucil in the USA.

78
Radish

E xtract the juice of a radish and mix it into a paste with milk. This can be applied to the painful area to relieve the symptoms of hemorrhoids. Alternatively, you can drink the juice of a ripe radish, but do drink it with at least the same quantity of carrot or other juice.

79
Reinsertion

After making sure that your fingernails are filed short and smooth, you can try gently pushing hemorrhoids back into the anus. This should relieve most of the pain.

80
Rustyback Fern

This species of fern grows in Europe and has hairs that are orange/brown in colour, hence its name. It is a common treatment for hemorrhoids.

Crush a leaf and bring to the boil in a pint of water.

After simmering for a couple of minutes filter the liquid through a cloth and let it stand and ferment for several hours.

Drink a small glass two or three times per day.

81
St Johns Wort Oil

St Johns Wort is also known as Tiptons Weed or *Hypericum perforatum*. It is a yellow herb that is native to Europe.

It is often sold as cream. Its active ingredient is hypercin which is anti-inflammatory.

82
Senna

Senna is the name for a large genus of flowering plants which have been used medicinally for thousands of years.

Alexandrian Senna has been particularly popular as a laxative to counteract constipation and piles.

83
Sesame Seeds

Sesame is a flowering plant native to Africa and India. It is cultivated for its oil rich, edible seeds that are exceptionally rich in calcium copper iron magnesium and manganese.

It is used in Ayurvedic medicine for the treatment of hemorrhoids.

Take about 40g of seeds and boil in a litre of water until only a third of the liquid remains. Remove the seeds, mash them with butter and eat.

84
Sitz Bath

A sitz bath is a bath that enables the buttocks and hips to be covered by warm water. It relaxes the sphincter and increases blood flow to the area, promoting faster healing. It can provide relief from pain and itching.

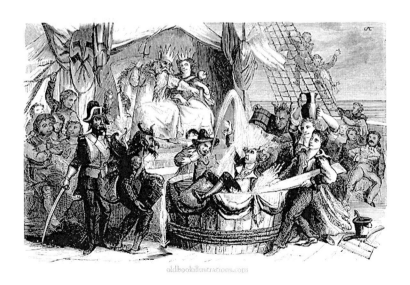

Ideally the water temperature is fairly hot for a 20 – 30 minute period whilst it is being used. You can buy a sitz bath that sits over a toilet, with a continuous flow of warm water overflowing into the toilet.

Some find it beneficial to add Epsom salts or aromatherapy oils. Or you can alternate hot and cold baths every few minutes. Dry the area well afterwards.

85
Slippery Elm

S lippery elm is a deciduous tree native to North America. The inner bark can be ground and mixed with water to make a gruel that is rich in nutrients. Alternatively it can be dried, ground into a powder, and made into a tea.

86
Soft Toilet Paper

N ot only will soft toilet paper be less likely to rub or inflame the affected are, it also requires less wipes, being more absorbent. Cleaning gently with a hypoallergenic soap and cool water ,and then patting dry, once a day is also desirable.

87
Sulphur

H istorically known as brimstone , and also called Sublimed Sulphur, it is used in homeopathy to relieve hemorrhoids.

88
Triphala

T riphala is an Ayurvedic, traditional Indian, treatment that literally means "three fruits". It is used to promote appetite and digestion. By relieving constipation and increasing the red blood cell count it helps treat hemorrhoids.

89
Turmeric

T urmeric is a plant of the ginger family native to tropical south Asia that is used in Ayurvedic practices to relieve hemorrhoids. It can be bought as a cream and applied.

90
Turnip

The juice of a turnip can be mixed with carrot juice and is said to relieve hemorrhoid pain.

91
Water

Most of us drink too little water. Drinking at least 8 large glasses a day is especially important for piles sufferers as it ensures that the body has sufficient moisture to aid digestion. Avoiding caffeine in tea and coffee can also help as caffeine is a diuretic.

92
White Leadwort

The Latin name is *Plumbago zeylanica*, and it is a herb native to India. The root is used in Ayurvedic medicine because it contains Plumbagin, an antiseptic that stimulates the central nervous system. It is dangerous in large quantities, so it is especially important to only use this under medical supervision.

93
White Oak Bark

The White Oak is a North American hardwood. It is known as an astringent and can tighten and strengthen vascular walls. You can steam or boil the bark and apply to the area or make it into a tea.

94
Witch Hazel

Witch hazel is a North American shrub that was widely used by Native Americans as a medicine. It is a strong anti-oxidant and astringent. It both soothes and shrinks the inflamed blood vessels.

95
Yam

Yam is also known by its Latin name of *Dioscorea*. It is a perennial vine cultivated in the subtropics. In Ayurvedic medicine it is used to make Karunai.

96
Yarrow

Yarrow is also known as Nosebleed Plant and *Achilea millefolium*. It is a herbaceous perennial plant native to the Northern Hemisphere.

It has been used for many centuries because of its astringent properties, particularly prevalent in its flowers. .

97
Yellow Dock

Yellow dock, also known as Curled Dock or *Rumex Crispus* is a perennial flowering plant native to Europe and Asia.

The root contains anthraquinones which stimulates bowel movements. It also has a substantial amount of tannins, an astringent which also helps treat hemorrhoids.

It has been used in Chinese medicine and more widely.

98
Yellow Sweet Clover

Yellow sweet clover is also known as Yellow Melilot or *Melilotus officinalis*. Native to Europe and Asia, it is now found throughout the world.

Herbalists use it to combat hemorrhoids as it reduces fluid retention in vein walls.

99
Yoga

Yoga is ideal for strengthening key muscles that eliminate the need for straining when going to the toilet and also reducing the pressure on the pelvic region generally.

If time is limited then the head stand pose is ideal.

Kneel on a mat, and then place your head on it. Keeping your hands behind your head, raise your legs. They don't need to be vertical if you can't manage that.

Maintain the position for up to 30 seconds and repeat daily. This will relieve the pressure from the pelvic and rectal area.

Alternatively try the candle pose.

Lay on your back, with your feet together and your hands at your sides. Bring your knees up to your chest.

Swing your hips up, bending your elbows to hold your back up with your hands. Keep your upper arms on the floor. Try to straighten your back and lift your legs up as vertically as possible.

Breathe deeply and hold the pose for 10-30 seconds. Lower your legs and back gently and slowly.

100
Yoghurt

Yoghurt is said by some to provide relief. It can be mixed with pomegranate juice and either coriander or ginger paste before being eaten.

It is a better source of protein and calcium than milk, cheese or cream if you suffer from hemorrhoids.

Yoghurt has few of the properties in other dairy products that can lead to constipation.

101
Zinc Oxide

Zinc oxide (or petroleum jelly) is much cheaper than many proprietary hemorrhoid creams. It can form a barrier over the hemorrhoids and reduce itching.

Zinc Oxide can be applied with a cotton wool ball to the affected area after it has been washed and dried well.

Some sufferers alternate using Witch Hazel (an astringent) with Zinc Oxide to provide relief.

08/10

DEMCO

LaVergne, TN USA
16 August 2010
193482LV00009B/154/P